SOMATIC EXERCISES FOR BEGINNERS

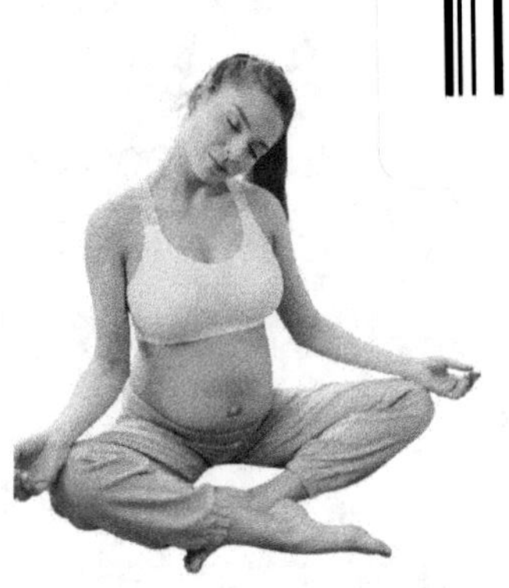

Discover the Joy of Somatic Movement: Gentle Exercises for Beginners to Enhance Body Awareness and Well-being

By

Lois Massy

TABLE OF CONTENTS

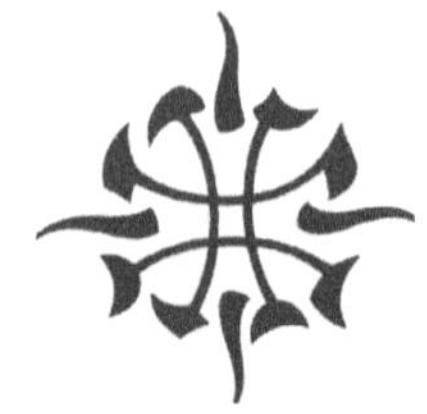

INTRODUCTION

Somatic exercises are a type of movement practice that focus on enhancing somatic awareness and promoting mind-body integration. The term "somatic" refers to the lived experience of the body, involving sensations, perceptions, and emotions. Somatic exercises aim to improve the quality of movement, release muscular tension, and restore optimal functioning of the body.

WHAT ARE SOMATIC EXERCISES?

Somatic exercises are a series of gentle and slow movements designed to bring attention to the internal sensations and patterns of tension held within the body. Unlike traditional exercise modalities that often involves repetitive and externalized movements, somatic exercises emphasize internal awareness and conscious control of movement.

These exercises draw inspiration from various disciplines such as somatics, Feldenkrais Method, Alexander Technique, and Body-Mind Centering. They are based on the principle that the brain and nervous system have the capacity to reprogram and reorganize muscular patterns, leading to improved posture, movement efficiency, and overall well-being.

Somatic exercises involve exploring different movement sequences and variations, often performed in a slow, deliberate, and mindful manner. They encourage individuals to pay attention to subtle sensations, release unnecessary muscular tension, and develop a deeper connection with their bodies.

BENEFITS OF SOMATIC EXERCISE

Engaging in somatic exercises can offer numerous benefits for individuals of all ages and physical abilities. These exercises focus on enhancing body awareness, promoting mind-body integration, and improving overall well-being. Here are some of the key benefits of somatic exercise:

1. Increased Body Awareness: Somatic exercises help individuals develop a heightened sense of body awareness. Through slow and mindful movements, practitioners learn to pay attention to subtle sensations and internal cues. This increased body awareness allows individuals to recognize and understand their habitual movement patterns, postural imbalances, and areas of tension or discomfort.

2. Improved Movement Efficiency: Somatic exercises aim to optimize movement patterns and improve neuromuscular coordination. By releasing unnecessary muscular tension and restoring balanced movement, individuals can enhance movement efficiency and reduce effort in daily activities. This can result in improved performance in sports, dance, and other physical activities.

3. Enhanced Flexibility and Range of Motion: Somatic exercises often incorporate gentle stretching and mobilization of joints. By moving through a full range of motion with awareness and relaxation, individuals can gradually increase their flexibility and improve joint mobility. This can lead to greater ease and fluidity of movement.

4. Pain Relief and Tension Reduction: Somatic exercises can be effective in alleviating chronic muscular pain and tension. By addressing underlying patterns of muscular contraction and releasing excessive tension, these exercises help individuals experience relief from conditions such as back pain, neck and shoulder tension, and muscle stiffness. Somatic exercises can also help individuals manage stress-related muscle tension and reduce the risk of repetitive strain injuries.

5. Stress Reduction and Relaxation: Somatic exercises often incorporate elements of mindfulness and relaxation techniques. By practicing slow, intentional movements and focusing on the present moment, individuals can experience a sense of calm and relaxation. This can help reduce stress levels, improve sleep quality, and promote overall mental well-being.

6. Improved Posture and Alignment: Somatic exercises can help individuals improve their postural alignment and body mechanics. By developing awareness of postural habits and releasing excessive muscular tension, individuals can achieve a more balanced and aligned posture. This can reduce the risk of postural imbalances, such as forward head posture or rounded shoulders, which can lead to pain and musculoskeletal issues.

7. Mind-Body Integration: Somatic exercises emphasize the connection between the mind and body. By engaging in mindful movement and cultivating body awareness, individuals can develop a deeper understanding of the interplay between their physical sensations, emotions, and mental states. This mind-body integration can lead to a greater sense of self-awareness, improved emotional well-being, and a more holistic approach to health and wellness.

GETTING STARTED: PRECAUTIONS AND CONSIDERATIONS

Before starting a somatic exercise practice, it's important to consider a few precautions and factors:

1. Consult with a Healthcare Professional: If you have any pre-existing medical conditions, injuries, or physical limitations, it's advisable to consult with a healthcare professional before beginning somatic exercises. They can provide personalized guidance and ensure that the exercises are suitable for your specific needs and abilities.

2. Start Slow and Gradual: Somatic exercises are typically gentle and slow-paced. It's important to start with basic movements and gradually progress as your body adapts and becomes more familiar with the exercises. Rushing into complex movements or pushing beyond your comfort level can increase the risk of injury.

3. Listen to Your Body: Pay attention to your body's signals and limitations during somatic exercises. Avoid any movements that cause pain or discomfort. Remember that somatic exercises are meant to be performed with a sense of ease and relaxation, so adjust the intensity and range of motion based on what feels comfortable for you.

4. Practice Mindfulness and Presence: Somatic exercises involve cultivating mindful awareness of your body and its sensations. Approach the exercises with a sense of curiosity, non-judgment, and presence. Focus on the quality of movement and the sensory experience rather than striving for perfection or external goals.

5. Personalize Your Practice: Somatic exercises can be tailored to your individual needs and goals. Modify the exercises to accommodate your body's unique abilities and limitations. Seek guidance from a qualified somatic practitioner or instructor who can provide personalized recommendations and adjustments.

Remember, somatic exercises are a journey of self-discovery and self-care. Consistency and patience are key. As you develop a regular somatic exercise practice, you may gradually experience the benefits of increased body awareness, improved movement efficiency, pain relief, stress reduction, enhanced posture, and a deeper mind-body connection.

Chapter 1

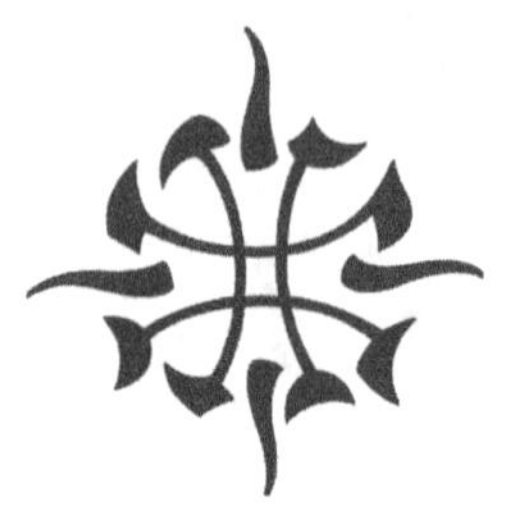

Basic Principles of Somatic Exercises

Somatic exercises are guided by several fundamental principles that form the foundation of this movement practice. These principles help individuals develop a deeper understanding of their bodies, improve movement patterns, and promote mind-body integration. Here are some of the basic principles of somatic exercises:

1. Sensory Awareness: Sensory awareness is a key principle in somatic exercises. It involves cultivating a heightened perception of internal sensations and bodily experiences. By paying attention to the subtle sensations and feedback from the body, individuals can develop a greater understanding of their movement patterns, areas of tension, and overall body condition. Sensory awareness allows for a more nuanced and informed approach to movement, leading to improved body control and a more refined sense of proprioception.

2. Slow and Mindful Movements: Somatic exercises are typically performed at a slow and deliberate pace. This deliberate slowness allows individuals to tune in to the nuances of their movements, explore their range of motion, and experience the sensory feedback from each movement. Slow and mindful movements promote a deeper mind-body connection, enhance body awareness, and facilitate the rewiring of neurological pathways involved in movement patterns.

3. Voluntary Muscle Control: Somatic exercises emphasize voluntary muscle control, which involves consciously engaging and releasing specific muscles during movement. This principle allows individuals to become aware of patterns of unnecessary muscular tension and learn to release it consciously. By developing voluntary control over muscles, individuals can improve movement efficiency, reduce unnecessary effort, and prevent chronic muscle tension.

4. Non-Habitual Movement Exploration: Somatic exercises often involve exploring movements that deviate from habitual patterns. By introducing novel movement sequences and variations, individuals can break free from limiting movement patterns and expand their movement repertoire. Non-habitual movement exploration helps to rewire the brain-body connections and promotes neuroplasticity, allowing for greater adaptability, creativity, and freedom in movement.

5. Body-Mind Integration: Somatic exercises emphasize the integration of the body and mind. They recognize that the mind and body are interconnected and that our thoughts, emotions, and beliefs can influence our physical experiences. By cultivating a conscious and intentional relationship between the mind and body during somatic exercises, individuals can develop a deeper mind-body connection. This integration can lead to a sense of wholeness, improved emotional well-being, and a greater sense of self-awareness.

Mind-Body Connection

The mind-body connection is a central aspect of somatic exercises. It refers to the reciprocal relationship between our thoughts, emotions, and bodily experiences. Somatic exercises recognize that our mental and emotional states can influence our physical well-being, and vice versa.

When practicing somatic exercises, individuals are encouraged to bring their attention to the present moment and to develop a conscious awareness of their bodily sensations, movements, and breath. This focus on the present moment helps to cultivate mindfulness and deepen the mind-body connection.

By developing a stronger mind-body connection, individuals can gain insights into the ways in which their thoughts, emotions, and stress levels impact their physical well-being. They can also learn to use movement and body awareness as tools for managing stress, reducing tension, and promoting overall well-being.

The mind-body connection in somatic exercises is not limited to mental and emotional influences on the body. It also acknowledges the role of the body in influencing our mental and emotional states. For example, by releasing physical tension and promoting relaxation through somatic exercises, individuals can experience a reduction in stress and an improvement in their emotional state.

Overall, the mind-body connection in somatic exercises emphasizes the holistic nature of our well-being and highlights the importance of addressing both physical and mental aspects of health. By integrating the mind and body in our movement practice, we can enhance our overall well-being and develop a deeper understanding of ourselves.

1. Embodied Mindfulness: Somatic exercises incorporate principles of mindfulness, which involves bringing non-judgmental awareness to the present moment. This mindful approach extends beyond the mental realm and includes a deep connection with the body. By cultivating embodied mindfulness during somatic exercises, individuals can develop a richer and more holistic experience of their physical sensations, emotions, and thoughts.

2. Emotional Release and Regulation: Somatic exercises can facilitate emotional release and regulation.

The body often holds onto unresolved emotions, stress, and trauma, which can manifest as muscular tension and discomfort. By engaging in somatic exercises and bringing awareness to the body, individuals can create a safe space to explore and release these stored emotions. This process supports emotional healing, stress reduction, and improved emotional well-being.

3. Body Language and Non-Verbal Communication: The body communicates information through non-verbal cues such as posture, gestures, and facial expressions. Somatic exercises can enhance our understanding of body language and non-verbal communication. By developing greater body awareness and sensitivity, individuals can become more attuned to their own non-verbal cues and the cues of others. This can foster better communication, empathy, and connection in personal and professional relationships.

4. Stress Reduction and Relaxation Response: Somatic exercises promote the activation of the relaxation response, which is the body's natural counterbalance to the stress response. Engaging in slow, mindful movements and deepening the mind-body connection activates the parasympathetic nervous system, leading to reduced stress levels, lowered heart rate, and increased relaxation. Regular practice of somatic exercises can help individuals manage stress more effectively and promote a greater sense of calm and well-being.

5. Body Mapping and Body Image: Somatic exercises facilitate a deeper understanding and acceptance of our bodies through body mapping. Body mapping involves exploring and refining our internal perception of our bodies, including the location and quality of sensations, movement patterns, and alignment. By developing a more accurate and nuanced body map, individuals can cultivate a healthier body image and a greater sense of embodiment.

6. Proception and Self-Regulation: Somatic exercises enhance interoception, which is the ability to perceive and interpret internal bodily sensations. Interoception plays a crucial role in self-regulation, allowing individuals to recognize and respond to their physiological needs, such as hunger, fatigue, and stress. By honing interoceptive skills through somatic exercises, individuals can develop a deeper connection with their bodies and make informed choices that support their overall well-being.

7. **Resilience and Self-Empowerment:** The mind-body connection cultivated through somatic exercises contributes to resilience and self-empowerment. By developing a greater awareness of our bodily sensations, movement patterns, and emotional states, we can recognize the early signs of stress or discomfort. This awareness empowers us to take proactive steps to address our needs, make healthier choices, and build resilience in the face of challenges.

The mind-body connection is a dynamic and multifaceted aspect of somatic exercises. By nurturing this connection, individuals can experience profound shifts in their physical well-being, emotional balance, and overall quality of life.

Sensory Awareness

Sensory awareness is a fundamental principle of somatic exercises. It involves developing a heightened perception and conscious attention to the various sensory experiences within the body. By cultivating sensory awareness, individuals can deepen their understanding of their own bodies and gain valuable insights into their movement patterns, areas of tension, and overall physical well-being.

1. Internal Sensations: Somatic exercises encourage individuals to pay attention to the internal sensations of their bodies. This includes noticing subtle cues such as muscle tension, joint mobility, breath patterns, and the quality of movement. By attuning to these sensations, individuals can develop a more nuanced understanding of their bodies and make informed choices about movement and posture.

2. Proprioception: Proprioception refers to the body's ability to sense its position, movement, and orientation in space. Somatic exercises help to refine and enhance proprioceptive abilities by focusing on the sensory feedback from the muscles, joints, and connective tissues during movement. This heightened proprioception allows individuals to move with greater precision, coordination, and efficiency.

3. Kinesthetic Awareness: Kinesthetic awareness involves perceiving and understanding the body's movement in relation to the surrounding environment. Somatic exercises facilitate the development of kinesthetic awareness by encouraging individuals to explore movement in different planes, directions, and speeds. This helps to refine spatial awareness, body coordination, and the ability to adapt to various physical contexts.

4. Interoception: Interoception refers to the perception and interpretation of internal bodily sensations, such as hunger, thirst, fatigue, and emotional states. Somatic exercises promote interoceptive awareness by guiding individuals to notice and respond to the subtle changes in their internal landscape during movement. This deepened interoception enhances self-regulation, emotional well-being, and the ability to make choices that support overall health.

SLOW AND GENTLE MOVEMENTS

Somatic exercises are characterized by slow and gentle movements. This deliberate pace is essential for fostering body awareness, allowing individuals to tune in to the sensory feedback and subtle nuances of their movements. Here's why slow and gentle movements are emphasized in somatic exercises:

1. Mind-Body Connection: Slow movements facilitate a deeper mind-body connection. By moving slowly and intentionally, individuals can develop a heightened awareness of their bodies, including the sensations, tensions, and limitations they may encounter. This conscious and deliberate approach promotes a more integrated experience of movement, fostering a greater connection between the mind and body.

2. Sensory Feedback: Slow movements enable individuals to receive and process the sensory feedback from their bodies more effectively. By moving at a slower pace, individuals can discern the nuances of muscle activation, joint mobility, and body alignment. This sensory feedback informs their movement choices and allows for adjustments that optimize movement patterns and reduce unnecessary tension.

3. Muscle Relaxation: Slow and gentle movements promote relaxation and release of muscular tension. By moving slowly, individuals have more time to notice areas of tension and consciously relax those muscles. This relaxation response helps to reduce chronic muscular tension, improve flexibility, and restore balanced muscle tone.

4. Neural Rewiring: Slow and deliberate movements support the rewiring of neural pathways involved in movement patterns. By repetitively engaging in slow and controlled movements, individuals can retrain their nervous system, breaking free from habitual patterns and establishing new, more efficient movement patterns. This neural rewiring enhances motor control, coordination, and overall movement efficiency.

5. Injury Prevention: Slow and gentle movements reduce the risk of injury during exercise. By moving slowly, individuals can maintain greater control and stability throughout the range of motion, minimizing the chances of strain, sprain, or overexertion. This cautious approach allows individuals to explore their limits and boundaries safely, gradually expanding their movement capacity over time.

By emphasizing sensory awareness and incorporating slow and gentle movements, somatic exercises provide a unique approach to movement and body awareness. This intentional and mindful practice allows individuals to develop a deeper understanding of their bodies, optimize movement patterns, and promote overall well-being.

Here's an additional information on sensory awareness and slow and gentle movements:

Sensory Awareness:

1. Body Mapping: Somatic exercises often involve body mapping, which is the process of developing a detailed internal representation of one's body. By paying attention to subtle sensations and exploring the body's various regions, individuals can create a more accurate and nuanced body map. This awareness of one's body helps in improving posture, movement quality, and overall body coordination.

2. Tension Release: Sensory awareness in somatic exercises allows individuals to identify areas of tension and discomfort in their bodies. By bringing attention to these areas and consciously releasing tension, individuals can promote relaxation, reduce chronic muscle tension, and alleviate pain. This process of tension release supports overall well-being and enhances movement efficiency.

3. Breath Awareness: Somatic exercises often emphasize breath awareness as a key component of sensory awareness. By paying attention to the breath, individuals can observe its quality, depth, and rhythm during movement. Conscious breathing can help regulate the nervous system, promote relaxation, and enhance body-mind integration.

4. Mindfulness in Daily Life: Somatic exercises cultivate sensory awareness not only during exercise sessions but also in daily life. By integrating sensory awareness practices into everyday activities, individuals can develop a greater connection with their bodies and a heightened sense of presence. This mindfulness in daily life supports overall well-being and enables individuals to make conscious choices that promote physical and mental health.

Slow and Gentle Movements:

1. Motor Control and Coordination: Slow and gentle movements in somatic exercises enhance motor control and coordination. By moving slowly, individuals can focus on the quality and precision of their movements, activating the appropriate muscles and joints. This deliberate control and coordination translate into improved movement patterns, balance, and stability.

2. Deepening Body Awareness: Slow movements allow individuals to deepen their body awareness and explore subtle sensations. By moving at a slower pace, individuals can notice and discern the intricate feedback from their bodies, such as muscle activation, joint alignment, and weight distribution. This heightened body awareness supports a more refined and conscious approach to movement.

3. Mindful Exploration: Slow and gentle movements provide an opportunity for mindful exploration of the body's capabilities and limitations. Individuals can observe how different movements feel, how they affect different parts of the body, and how they influence their overall well-being. This mindful exploration promotes a sense of curiosity, self-discovery, and a deeper connection with the body.

4. Stress Reduction and Relaxation: Slow movements in somatic exercises promote relaxation and stress reduction. By engaging in slow and gentle movements, individuals activate the parasympathetic nervous system, triggering the relaxation response. This physiological shift leads to reduced stress levels, improved sleep, and a greater sense of calm and well-being.

5. Rehabilitation and Injury Prevention: Slow and gentle movements are often utilized in rehabilitation settings to aid in injury recovery. By moving at a controlled pace, individuals can gradually rebuild strength, flexibility, and mobility without excessively straining injured tissues. Slow movements also help improve body alignment, joint stability, and proprioceptive feedback, reducing the risk of future injuries.

Sensory awareness and slow gentle movements are integral to somatic exercises. By honing these practices, individuals can cultivate a deeper connection with their bodies, enhance movement quality, reduce stress, and promote overall well-being.

BREATH AWARENESS

Breath awareness is a fundamental aspect of somatic exercises and mindfulness practices. It involves directing attention to the breath and cultivating a conscious, non-judgmental awareness of its flow, depth, and rhythm. Here's more information on breath awareness and its benefits:

1. Mind-Body Connection: Breath awareness deepens the mind-body connection by bringing attention to the present moment and the sensations of the breath within the body. By focusing on the breath, individuals can anchor themselves in the present, fostering a sense of embodied awareness and promoting a greater connection between the mind and body.

2. Stress Reduction: Breath awareness is a powerful tool for stress reduction. When individuals are stressed, their breath tends to become shallow and rapid. By consciously observing and regulating the breath, individuals can activate the body's relaxation response, triggering a state of calm and reducing stress levels. Deep, slow breaths can help regulate the autonomic nervous system, promoting a sense of relaxation and well-being.

3. Emotional Regulation: The breath is closely linked to emotions, and breath awareness can support emotional regulation. By paying attention to the breath, individuals can notice how emotions manifest as changes in the breath pattern. For example, anxiety often correlates with shallow, rapid breaths, while relaxation is associated with slow, deep breaths. By observing these patterns, individuals can use breath awareness to modulate their emotional states and promote emotional balance.

4. Body-Mind Integration: Breath awareness facilitates body-mind integration by allowing individuals to observe how the breath affects the body and vice versa. By consciously regulating the breath, individuals can influence their physiological responses, such as heart rate, blood pressure, and muscle tension. This integration of breath and body supports overall well-being and helps individuals respond to stressors in a more balanced and adaptive manner.

5. Increased Energy and Vitality: Deep, diaphragmatic breathing through breath awareness can enhance oxygenation and increase energy levels. By taking slow, deep breaths, individuals can improve the oxygen exchange in the lungs, nourishing the body's cells and tissues. This increased oxygenation promotes vitality, mental clarity, and a sense of invigoration.

6. Mindfulness and Presence: Breath awareness is a core practice in mindfulness meditation. By focusing on the breath, individuals anchor their attention to the present moment, cultivating mindfulness and presence. The breath serves as a focal point for attention, helping individuals develop a non-judgmental awareness of their thoughts, emotions, and bodily sensations as they arise and pass away.

7. Relaxation and Sleep Improvement: Practicing breath awareness before sleep can promote relaxation and improve sleep quality. By engaging in slow, deep breaths and consciously releasing tension, individuals can calm the nervous system, reduce racing thoughts, and prepare the body for restful sleep. This practice can be particularly helpful for individuals experiencing insomnia or difficulty falling asleep.

Breath awareness is a versatile and accessible practice that can be integrated into various aspects of life. By cultivating a conscious relationship with the breath, individuals can enhance their well-being, reduce stress, and develop a greater sense of presence and self-awareness.

1. Pranayama: Breath awareness is a fundamental component of pranayama, a yogic practice that involves conscious breath control. Pranayama techniques emphasize specific breath patterns, such as deep belly breathing, alternate nostril breathing, or extended exhalations. These techniques can have various effects on the body and mind, including energizing, calming, or balancing.

2. Body-Mind Integration: Breath awareness promotes the integration of the body and mind by fostering a deeper understanding of the body's responses and sensations. By observing the breath, individuals can notice how it affects different areas of the body, such as the chest, abdomen, and diaphragm. This awareness helps individuals develop a more embodied experience and make conscious choices that support their physical and mental well-being.

3. Emotional Awareness and Regulation: Breath awareness allows individuals to observe the link between the breath and emotions. By paying attention to the breath during different emotional states, individuals can notice patterns, such as shallow breathing during anxiety or deep, relaxed breathing during calmness. This awareness provides valuable insight into emotional states and offers an opportunity to regulate and balance emotions through intentional breath work.

4. Mindful Stress Management: Breath awareness is an effective tool for managing stress and promoting relaxation. By focusing on the breath, individuals can shift their attention away from stressful thoughts and into the present moment. Deep, slow breaths activate the body's relaxation response, helping to reduce stress hormones, lower heart rate, and induce a sense of calm and well-being.

5. Improved Concentration and Focus: Breath awareness enhances concentration and focus. By directing attention to the breath, individuals develop a single-pointed focus that can improve cognitive performance and productivity. The rhythmic nature of the breath serves as an anchor, allowing individuals to bring their attention back to the present moment whenever the mind wanders.

6. Mind-Body Healing: Breath awareness is often incorporated into mind-body healing practices. By consciously engaging with the breath, individuals can support the body's natural healing processes and facilitate self-regulation. Breath work can be used as a complementary practice alongside other therapeutic modalities to promote physical, mental, and emotional well-being.

7. Breathwork Techniques: Breath awareness can be further explored through specific breathwork techniques. These techniques involve intentional manipulation of the breath to achieve specific outcomes. Examples include deep belly breathing, box breathing (equal inhales, holds, exhales), or rapid breaths for energizing purposes. These techniques can be practiced during designated breathwork sessions or integrated into daily life as a tool for self-regulation and well-being.

Breath awareness is a versatile practice that can be adapted to individual needs and preferences. By incorporating breath awareness into daily life or dedicating specific time for breath-focused practices, individuals can enhance their overall well-being, emotional regulation, and experience a deeper sense of connection with themselves and the present moment.

Chapter 2

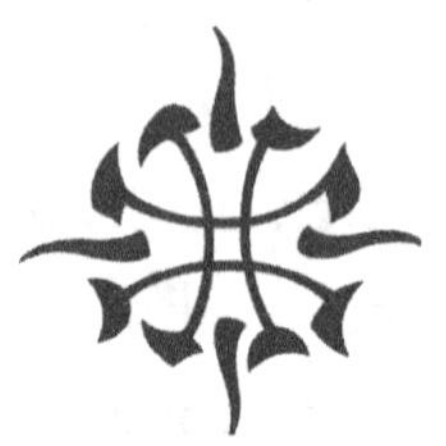

Preparing for Somatic Exercises

CREATING A SAFE AND COMFORTABLE SPACE

Creating a safe and comfortable space is crucial when preparing for somatic exercises. Here are some key considerations to ensure an optimal environment:

1. Clear the Space: Start by clearing any clutter or obstacles from the area where you'll be practicing somatic exercises. This helps create a safe and unobstructed space for movement. Remove any furniture or objects that may hinder your movements and create a clear path.

2. Adequate Lighting: Ensure that the space is well-lit to avoid any accidents or strain on your eyes. Natural light is ideal, but if that's not possible, use a combination of overhead and task lighting to provide sufficient illumination.

3. Temperature and Ventilation: Maintain a comfortable temperature in the room to support relaxation and ease of movement. Ensure proper ventilation to keep the air fresh and conducive to deep breathing. Consider opening windows or using fans if necessary.

4. Non-Slip Surface: Choose a surface that is firm and non-slip to prevent accidents or injuries. If practicing on a hard floor, you may want to use a non-slip mat or yoga mat for added comfort and stability.

5. Quiet and Peaceful Environment: Minimize distractions and create a quiet and peaceful atmosphere for your somatic exercises. Turn off or silence any electronic devices, reduce background noise, and choose a time when you're less likely to be interrupted.

6. Privacy: Find a space where you can have privacy and feel comfortable. This allows you to fully engage in the somatic exercises without self-consciousness or distractions. Close the doors and let others know that you need uninterrupted time during your practice.

7. Supportive Props: Depending on the specific somatic exercises you'll be doing, you may need props such as pillows, blankets, or yoga blocks for support and comfort. Have these props nearby and easily accessible.

8. Comfortable Clothing: Wear loose, comfortable clothing that allows for unrestricted movement. Avoid tight or restrictive clothing that may hinder your ability to fully engage in the exercises.

9. Mindful Presence: Before starting your somatic exercises, take a few moments to center yourself and cultivate a sense of mindful presence. Set an intention for your practice and create a mental space for focused awareness and self-exploration.

Remember, the goal is to create a safe, comfortable, and supportive environment that allows you to fully engage in the somatic exercises and deepen your mind-body connection. By preparing your space mindfully, you can enhance the effectiveness and enjoyment of your somatic practice.

Clothing:

- Choose loose, comfortable clothing that allows for unrestricted movement. Opt for materials that are breathable and stretchy, such as cotton or moisture-wicking fabrics.

- Avoid clothing with restrictive waistbands, tight sleeves, or excessive layers that may limit your range of motion.

- Dress in layers so you can adjust your clothing according to your body temperature during the practice.

- Consider wearing form-fitting or supportive undergarments to ensure comfort and ease of movement.

Equipment:

- The beauty of somatic exercises is that they often require minimal equipment. However, depending on the specific exercises or techniques you'll be practicing, you may find the following items helpful:

- Yoga mat or exercise mat: Provides cushioning and support for exercises done on the floor.

- Blankets or cushions: Can be used to support different parts of the body or provide comfort during seated or lying-down exercises.

- Yoga blocks or straps: These props can assist with modifications or provide support when needed.

- Resistance bands or balls: These tools can be used to add resistance or assist with certain movements.

When choosing equipment, consider your specific needs, preferences, and the guidance of your somatic exercise instructor, if applicable.

WARM-UP AND STRETCHING FOR SOMATIC EXERCISES

Warm-up:

- Before starting somatic exercises, it's important to warm up your body to increase circulation, prepare the muscles and joints, and prevent injuries. Here are some ideas for a warm-up routine:

- Begin with some light cardiovascular activity like brisk walking, jumping jacks, or marching in place for a few minutes.

- Perform dynamic stretches that involve gentle movements through a full range of motion. Examples include arm circles, leg swings, shoulder rolls, and gentle twists.

- Gradually increase the intensity and range of motion as your body warms up, but avoid pushing yourself too hard during the warm-up phase.

Stretching:

- Somatic exercises often incorporate gentle stretching movements to release tension, increase flexibility, and promote a sense of relaxation. Here are some considerations for stretching during somatic exercises:

- Focus on gentle and mindful stretching rather than forceful or aggressive movements.

- Move slowly and smoothly, paying attention to the sensations in your body and avoiding any pain or discomfort.

- Choose stretches that target the areas of your body that feel tight or restricted, and hold each stretch for an appropriate duration (usually around 15-30 seconds).

- Breathe deeply and relax into the stretches, allowing any tension to melt away.

Remember, warming up and stretching are essential for preparing your body for somatic exercises and optimizing your performance. However, the specific warm-up and stretching routine may vary depending on the type of somatic exercises you'll be practicing and your individual needs. It's always a good idea to consult with a qualified somatic exercise instructor or healthcare professional for personalized guidance and recommendations.

Here's some additional information on clothing and equipment for somatic exercises, as well as warm-up and stretching:

Clothing and Equipment for Somatic Exercises:

Clothing:

- Opt for clothing that allows for a wide range of motion and does not restrict your movement.

Loose-fitting, breathable fabrics like cotton or moisture-wicking materials are ideal.

- Choose clothing that is comfortable and non-restrictive, allowing you to fully engage in the somatic exercises without discomfort.

- Consider wearing layers, especially if you'll be practicing in a space with varying temperatures. This allows you to adjust your clothing as needed to maintain your comfort.

Equipment:

- Somatic exercises typically do not require much equipment, but there may be certain tools or props that can enhance your practice. Here are a few examples:

  - Yoga mat or exercise mat: Provides a comfortable and supportive surface for floor-based exercises.

  - Blankets or bolsters: Can be used to support different body parts, enhance relaxation, or provide cushioning during seated or lying-down positions.

  - Foam roller: Can be used for self-massage and releasing tension in specific muscle groups.

- Yoga blocks or straps: These props can assist with modifications or help you achieve proper alignment in certain poses or movements.

- Resistance bands: Can be used to add resistance and challenge to exercises, helping to strengthen muscles and improve flexibility.

The specific equipment you choose will depend on your individual needs, preferences, and the guidance of your somatic exercise instructor, if you have one.

Warm-up and Stretching for Somatic Exercises:

Warm-up:

- Prior to engaging in somatic exercises, it's important to warm up your body to increase blood flow, raise your core body temperature, and prepare your muscles and joints for movement. Here are some warm-up ideas:

- Begin with some light aerobic exercises like jogging in place, jumping jacks, or cycling on a stationary bike for about 5-10 minutes.

- Incorporate dynamic movements that gently mobilize the major joints of your body. Examples include arm swings, leg swings, hip circles, and shoulder rolls.

- Gradually increase the intensity and range of motion of your warm-up exercises, but avoid pushing yourself to the point of fatigue or discomfort.

Stretching:

- Stretching is an integral part of somatic exercises as it helps to release tension, improve flexibility, and promote body awareness. Here are some considerations for stretching during somatic exercises:

- Prioritize gentle, controlled stretching movements over forceful or aggressive stretches.

- Move slowly and mindfully through each stretch, paying attention to the sensations in your body and avoiding any pain.

- Focus on elongating the muscles and connective tissues involved in the specific somatic exercises you'll be practicing.

- Breathe deeply and relax into each stretch, allowing your body to gradually release tension and increase its range of motion.

It's important to note that the warm-up and stretching routines for somatic exercises may vary depending on the specific techniques you're practicing, your fitness level, and any individual considerations. It's always recommended to consult with a qualified somatic exercise instructor or healthcare professional for personalized guidance and to ensure you're performing the warm-up and stretching exercises safely and effectively.

Chapter 3

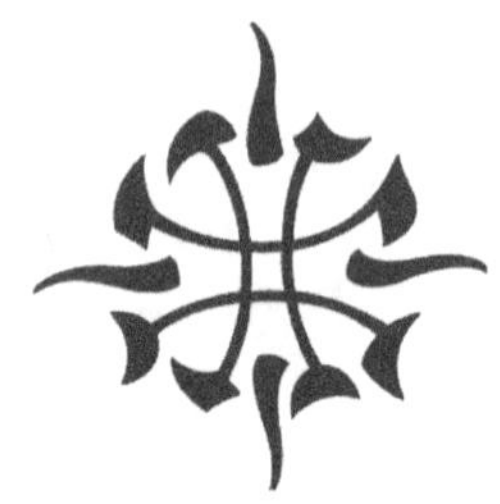

Somatic Exercises for the Neck and Shoulders

NECK ROLLS

The neck and shoulders are common areas where tension and discomfort can accumulate due to factors like poor posture, stress, and repetitive movements. Somatic exercises can help release tension and improve mobility in these areas. Here's an example of a somatic exercise for the neck and shoulders

Neck rolls are a gentle and effective somatic exercise to release tension and increase mobility in the neck and upper shoulders. Here's how to perform neck rolls:

1. Sit or stand in a comfortable position with your spine upright and your shoulders relaxed.

2. Take a few deep breaths to center yourself and bring your awareness to your neck and shoulders.

3. Begin by slowly tilting your head to the right, bringing your right ear towards your right shoulder. Keep your shoulders relaxed and avoid lifting or shrugging them.

4. Once your right ear is near your right shoulder, continue the movement by allowing your chin to drop towards your chest. Feel the gentle stretch along the left side of your neck.

5. Slowly roll your head to the left, bringing your left ear towards your left shoulder. Again, keep your shoulders relaxed and avoid lifting them.

6. Once your left ear is near your left shoulder, continue the movement by allowing your chin to rise towards the ceiling. Feel the gentle stretch along the right side of your neck.

7. Continue this smooth and gentle rolling motion, moving your head from side to side, allowing your ear to shoulder and chin to chest movements to flow together.

8. As you perform the neck rolls, pay attention to any areas of tension or resistance. Take your time and move with awareness, allowing the muscles to gradually release and relax.

9. Repeat the movement for several rounds, enjoying the fluidity and ease of the neck rolls.

10. After a few rounds, pause and take a moment to notice the effects of the exercise. Observe any changes in the sensation and mobility of your neck and shoulders.

It's important to approach neck rolls with gentleness and mindfulness. Avoid any sharp or jerky movements, and if you experience any pain or discomfort, reduce the range of motion or discontinue the exercise. Somatic exercises are meant to be done in a way that feels comfortable and safe for your body.

Remember, somatic exercises are most effective when practiced regularly and integrated into your daily routine. They can help you develop greater body awareness, release tension, and promote overall well-being in the neck and shoulder area.

Some additional information on somatic exercises for the neck and shoulders, including variations and tips for performing neck rolls:

In addition to neck rolls, there are other somatic exercises that can help release tension and improve mobility in the neck and shoulders. Here are a few examples:

1. Neck Tilts:

- Sit or stand with a tall spine and relaxed shoulders.

- Slowly tilt your head to the right, bringing your right ear towards your right shoulder.

- Hold the stretch for a few seconds, feeling the gentle stretch along the left side of your neck.

- Return your head to the center and repeat on the left side.

- Continue alternating sides for several repetitions, focusing on maintaining a smooth and controlled movement.

2. Shoulder Rolls:

- Sit or stand with your spine upright and your shoulders relaxed.

- Lift your shoulders towards your ears, then roll them back and down in a circular motion.

- Repeat the shoulder rolls in a fluid and controlled manner, allowing your shoulder blades to move freely.

- After several repetitions, reverse the direction of the shoulder rolls.

3. Neck and Shoulder Stretches:

- Sit or stand with a tall spine and relaxed shoulders.

- Bring your right arm up and over your head, placing your right hand on the left side of your head.

- Gently tilt your head to the right, feeling a stretch along the left side of your neck and shoulder.

- Hold the stretch for a few seconds, then switch sides and repeat.

- You can also perform a similar stretch by interlacing your fingers behind your head and gently pressing your head into your hands while maintaining an upright posture.

Variations and Modifications

- If you have limited mobility or discomfort in your neck and shoulders, you can modify the exercises to suit your needs. Reduce the range of motion, move more slowly, and listen to your body's signals to avoid any pain or strain.

- It's important to approach somatic exercises with gentleness and mindfulness. Avoid forceful or jerky movements, and prioritize smooth, controlled motions that promote relaxation and release of tension.

Tips for Performing Neck Rolls:

1. Move with Awareness: Pay close attention to the sensations in your neck and shoulders as you perform neck rolls. Notice areas of tension or restriction and aim to release and relax those areas with each movement.

2. Breathe Deeply: Deep, diaphragmatic breathing can help facilitate relaxation and enhance the benefits of the somatic exercises. Breathe in deeply through your nose, allowing your abdomen to expand, and exhale fully through your mouth, releasing any tension.

3. Take Breaks: If you find that your neck or shoulders become fatigued during the exercise, take short breaks or reduce the number of repetitions. It's important to respect your body's limits and avoid overexertion.

4. Regular Practice: Consistency is key when it comes to somatic exercises. Aim to incorporate these exercises into your daily routine to experience long-term benefits for your neck and shoulders.

Remember, somatic exercises are intended to be gentle, mindful, and performed within your comfort level. If you have any underlying medical conditions or concerns, it's always a good idea to consult with a healthcare professional before starting a new exercise routine.

SHOULDER ROLLS

Shoulder rolls are simple yet effective somatic exercises that can help release tension and improve mobility in the shoulder area. Here's how to perform shoulder rolls:

1. Stand or sit with your spine upright and your shoulders relaxed.

2. Begin by rolling your shoulders forward in a circular motion. Lift your shoulders up towards your ears, then roll them forward and down.

3. Continue the rolling motion, feeling the gentle stretch and release in your shoulder muscles.

4. After several forward rolls, reverse the direction. Roll your shoulders back, lifting them up towards your ears, then roll them back and down.

5. Perform the shoulder rolls in a slow, controlled, and fluid manner.

6. Focus on maintaining relaxation and ease throughout the movement. Avoid any forceful or jerky motions.

Neck and Shoulder Release

The neck and shoulder release exercise is a somatic movement that targets both the neck and shoulder muscles. Here's how to perform it:

1. Sit or stand with a tall spine and relaxed shoulders.

2. Take a deep breath in and, as you exhale, gently drop your chin towards your chest, allowing your head to relax forward.

3. Inhale and begin to roll your head to the right, bringing your right ear towards your right shoulder. Keep your shoulders relaxed and avoid lifting or shrugging them.

4. As you exhale, continue the movement by allowing your head to roll back, bringing your gaze towards the ceiling.

5. Inhale again and roll your head to the left, bringing your left ear towards your left shoulder.

6. Exhale and roll your head forward, returning to the starting position with your chin towards your chest.

7. Repeat the movement, flowing smoothly and slowly through the sequence.

8. As you perform the exercise, pay attention to any areas of tension or restriction in your neck and shoulders. Allow the movements to be gentle and exploratory, aiming to release and relax the muscles with each repetition.

9. Perform several rounds of the neck and shoulder release exercise, gradually increasing your range of motion and exploring different paths of movement.

Remember to move with awareness, focusing on the sensations in your body and avoiding any pain or discomfort. Modify the exercise as needed to suit your individual needs and limitations.

These somatic exercises can be incorporated into your daily routine to promote relaxation, release tension, and improve mobility in your neck and shoulder area. As always, if you have any underlying medical conditions or concerns, it's advisable to consult with a healthcare professional before starting a new exercise program.

Chapter 4

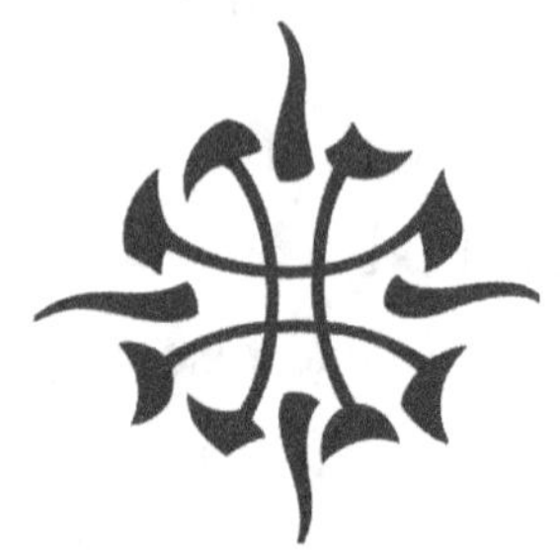

Somatic Exercises for the Back

SPINAL WAVE

The back is a common area where tension, stiffness, and discomfort can accumulate due to factors like poor posture, sedentary lifestyle, and stress. Somatic exercises can help release tension, improve mobility, and promote awareness of movement patterns in the back. One such exercise is the Spinal Wave.

The Spinal Wave is a somatic exercise that involves gently flexing and extending the spine to release tension and improve mobility. Here's how to perform the Spinal Wave:

1. Begin by standing with your feet hip-width apart and your knees slightly bent. Allow your arms to hang loosely by your sides.

2. Take a moment to bring your awareness to your back and spine. Notice any areas of tension or discomfort.

3. Start the movement by slowly tucking your tailbone under, rounding your spine, and allowing your head to drop forward. Imagine creating a C-shape with your spine.

4. Continue the movement by smoothly reversing the motion. Begin to slowly lift your tailbone, allowing your spine to unfurl, and bringing your head and chest up towards the ceiling. Imagine creating an arch with your spine.

5. As you perform this wave-like motion, aim for a smooth and controlled movement, articulating each vertebra in your spine.

6. Pay attention to any areas of tension or resistance as you move through the Spinal Wave. Allow the movement to be gentle and exploratory, focusing on releasing and relaxing the muscles in your back.

7. Perform several rounds of the Spinal Wave, gradually increasing the range of motion and exploring different pathways of movement.

8. As you become more comfortable with the exercise, you can synchronize your breath with the movement. Inhale as you round your spine and exhale as you extend your spine.

It's important to approach the Spinal Wave exercise with gentleness and mindfulness. Avoid any forceful or jerky movements, and if you experience any pain or discomfort, reduce the range of motion or discontinue the exercise. Somatic exercises are meant to be done in a way that feels comfortable and safe for your body.

The Spinal Wave exercise can be practiced regularly to promote relaxation, release tension, and improve mobility in your back. As always, if you have any underlying medical conditions or concerns, it's advisable to consult with a healthcare professional before starting a new exercise program.

Some additional information on somatic exercises for the back and the benefits of the Spinal Wave exercise:

Somatic Exercises for the Back:

In addition to the Spinal Wave, there are other somatic exercises that can help release tension and promote mobility in the back. Here are a few examples:

1. Cat-Cow Stretch:

- Begin on your hands and knees, with your wrists aligned under your shoulders and your knees under your hips.

- Inhale and gently arch your back, lifting your chest towards the ceiling, and allowing your belly to sink towards the floor. This is the cow position.

- Exhale and round your back, tucking your tailbone under, dropping your head, and drawing your belly button towards your spine. This is the cat position.

- Flow between the cat and cow positions, synchronizing your breath with the movements. Inhale for cow, exhale for cat.

- Continue the fluid motion for several rounds, focusing on releasing tension and promoting mobility in your spine.

2. Standing Forward Fold:

- Stand with your feet hip-width apart and soften your knees slightly.

- Slowly hinge forward at your hips, allowing your upper body to hang over your legs.

- Let your head and neck relax, and allow your arms to dangle towards the floor.

- You can gently sway from side to side or bend and straighten your knees to release tension in your back.

- Hold the stretch for several breaths, allowing your spine to lengthen and relax.

Benefits of the Spinal Wave Exercise:

The Spinal Wave exercise offers several benefits for the back and the body as a whole:

1. Releases Tension: The wave-like motion of the Spinal Wave helps to release tension and tightness in the muscles of the back. It can target areas of stiffness and promote a sense of relaxation.

2. Improves Mobility: By gently flexing and extending the spine, the Spinal Wave exercise helps to improve the mobility and flexibility of the back. It encourages a fuller range of motion and can enhance the overall function of the spine.

3. Enhances Body Awareness: Practicing the Spinal Wave exercise promotes body awareness and encourages a mindful connection with the movements of the back. It allows you to tune in to any areas of discomfort or restriction and work towards releasing them.

4. Promotes Spinal Health: The Spinal Wave exercise helps to maintain and promote the health of the spine. It encourages healthy movement patterns, improves circulation in the back, and can contribute to better posture and alignment.

It's important to note that somatic exercises like the Spinal Wave are intended to be gentle, mindful, and performed within your comfort level. Avoid any forceful or jerky movements, and listen to your body's signals to avoid pain or strain.

Incorporating somatic exercises like the Spinal Wave into your regular routine can help promote a healthier, more mobile, and relaxed back. Remember to consult with a healthcare professional if you have any underlying medical conditions or concerns before starting a new exercise program.

Cat-Cow Stretch

The Cat-Cow Stretch is a popular yoga exercise that helps to improve flexibility and mobility in the spine while stretching the back muscles. Here's how to perform it:

1. Start on your hands and knees, with your wrists aligned under your shoulders and your knees under your hips.

2. Inhale deeply and begin the movement by arching your back, dropping your belly towards the floor, and lifting your chest and gaze towards the ceiling. This is the Cow position.

3. As you exhale, round your spine upwards, tucking your chin towards your chest, and drawing your belly button towards your spine. This is the Cat position.

4. Flow smoothly between the Cow and Cat positions, moving with your breath. Inhale for Cow, exhale for Cat.

5. Repeat the movement for several rounds, paying attention to the sensations in your spine and allowing the movements to be fluid and gentle.

6. You can modify the exercise by incorporating gentle movements of your hips and pelvis to explore different angles and ranges of motion.

The Cat-Cow Stretch helps to release tension in the back, improves spinal flexibility, and can provide relief from back pain or stiffness. It also promotes body awareness and encourages a mindful connection with the movements of the spine.

PELVIC TILT

The Pelvic Tilt is a simple exercise that targets the muscles of the lower back, pelvis, and core. It helps to improve pelvic stability and flexibility. Here's how to perform it:

1. Lie on your back with your knees bent and your feet flat on the floor, hip-width apart.

2. Place your arms by your sides, palms facing down.

3. Inhale deeply, and as you exhale, engage your abdominal muscles and press your lower back gently into the floor.

4. Tilt your pelvis backward, flattening your lower back against the floor. You should feel a gentle contraction in your abdominal muscles.

5. Hold the position for a few seconds, maintaining a relaxed and steady breath.

6. Inhale, and as you exhale, release the tilt and allow your lower back to return to its natural curve.

7. Repeat the movement for several rounds, focusing on the gentle contraction and release of the lower back and abdominal muscles.

The Pelvic Tilt exercise helps to strengthen the core, improve pelvic stability, and promote proper alignment of the spine. It can be beneficial for individuals with lower back pain or those looking to improve their posture and strengthen their core muscles.

Both the Cat-Cow Stretch and the Pelvic Tilt are gentle and effective exercises that can be incorporated into your daily routine to promote a healthy and mobile back. As always, listen to your body, and if you have any underlying medical conditions or concerns, it's advisable to consult with a healthcare professional before starting a new exercise program.

The Back Twist, also known as the Seated Spinal Twist, is a yoga pose that helps to stretch and mobilize the muscles of the back, spine, and hips. It promotes spinal flexibility, releases tension, and improves overall mobility in the torso. Here's how to perform the Back Twist:

1. Start by sitting on the floor with your legs extended in front of you.

2. Bend your right knee and cross your right foot over your left leg, placing it flat on the floor next to your left knee.

3. Keep your left leg extended and your left foot flexed.

4. Inhale and lengthen your spine, sitting tall with your shoulders relaxed.

5. As you exhale, twist your torso to the right, placing your left elbow on the outside of your right knee. You can also bring your right hand behind you for support.

6. Maintain the length in your spine as you inhale, and with each exhale, deepen the twist by gently rotating your torso further to the right.

7. As you twist, keep your head in line with your spine or turn your gaze over your right shoulder, whichever feels comfortable for your neck.

8. Hold the twist for 30 seconds to 1 minute, breathing deeply and allowing your body to relax into the stretch.

9. To release the twist, inhale and slowly unwind your torso back to the center.

10. Repeat the twist on the other side, crossing your left foot over your right leg and twisting to the left.

It's important to approach the Back Twist with mindfulness and listen to your body's limits. Avoid forcing the twist or experiencing any pain or discomfort. Modify the pose as needed by using props like a bolster or blanket under your hips for support.

The Back Twist provides a gentle and effective stretch for the back, spine, and hips. Regular practice can help improve spinal mobility, alleviate back tension, and promote a sense of relaxation and well-being. As always, if you have any underlying medical conditions or concerns, it's advisable to consult with a healthcare professional before starting a new exercise program.

Some additional information about the Back Twist (Seated Spinal Twist) and its benefits:

Benefits of the Back Twist

1. Spinal Mobility: The Back Twist helps to improve flexibility and mobility in the spine. The twisting motion targets the muscles, ligaments, and connective tissues along the back, promoting a greater range of motion and enhancing overall spinal health.

2. Release of Tension: The twisting action in the Back Twist helps to release tension and tightness in the back muscles. It can relieve stiffness and discomfort caused by sedentary lifestyles, poor posture, or stress, providing a sense of relaxation and relief.

3. Improved Digestion: The twisting motion of the Back Twist stimulates the abdominal organs, including the digestive system. This can help to improve digestion, relieve bloating or discomfort, and promote overall digestive health.

4. Increased Energy Flow: Twisting poses in yoga are believed to help balance and stimulate the flow of energy throughout the body. The Back Twist can help to open up energy pathways and promote a sense of revitalization and well-being.

5. Stretching of Hips and Shoulders: Along with the back and spine, the Back Twist also stretches and opens the hips and shoulders. This can be particularly beneficial for individuals who spend long hours sitting or have tightness in these areas.

Tips for Practicing the Back Twist

1. Warm-up: It's recommended to warm up the body before practicing the Back Twist. Gentle movements like cat-cow stretches or seated forward bends can help prepare the spine and hips for the twist.

2. Modify as Needed: If you have any existing back or hip injuries or limitations, it's important to modify the pose accordingly. You can use props like bolsters, blankets, or blocks to support your body and make the pose more accessible.

3. Engage the Core: To enhance the twist and protect the lower back, engage your core muscles throughout the pose. This can help stabilize the spine and maintain proper alignment.

4. Breathe Mindfully: As you move into the Back Twist, focus on deep, steady breaths. Inhale to lengthen your spine, and exhale to deepen the twist. The breath can help you find relaxation and create more space in the body.

5. Gradual Progression: Over time, you can gradually deepen the twist as your body becomes more flexible and comfortable in the pose. However, always listen to your body's signals and avoid pushing beyond your limits.

The Back Twist is a versatile and beneficial exercise that can be practiced on its own or as part of a broader yoga practice. It can be done in the comfort of your own home or in a yoga class setting. Remember to honor your body's needs and consult with a healthcare professional if you have any concerns or pre-existing conditions.

Chapter 5

Somatic Exercises for the Hips and Pelvis

HIP CIRCLES

Hip circles are a type of somatic exercise that can help release tension and promote mobility in the hips and pelvis. They involve moving the hip joints in circular motions, which can improve the range of motion, increase circulation, and relieve stiffness in this area. Here's how to perform hip circles:

1. Stand with your feet hip-width apart and relax your arms by your sides.

2. Gently engage your core muscles to support your posture throughout the exercise.

3. Begin by shifting your weight onto your right leg while keeping your left leg relaxed.

4. Slowly start to make circular motions with your hips in a clockwise direction. Imagine drawing a circle with your hips.

5. As you move your hips in a circle, let the movement be fluid and relaxed. Avoid forcing the range of motion or creating any discomfort.

6. Gradually increase the size of the hip circles, exploring the full range of motion available to you.

7. After several circles in one direction, switch to counterclockwise circles.

8. Repeat the hip circles for several rounds, allowing your hips to move freely and naturally.

9. Take deep breaths as you perform the exercise, inhaling as you move forward in the circle and exhaling as you move backward.

10. After completing the desired number of circles, return to a neutral standing position and take a moment to notice any changes in your hips and pelvis.

Some tips to keep in mind while performing hip circles:

- Start with small circles and gradually increase the size as your range of motion improves.

- Keep the movement gentle and fluid, avoiding any jerking or abrupt motions.

- Focus on relaxing the muscles of the hips and pelvis throughout the exercise.

- Pay attention to any sensations or areas of tension, and adjust the movement accordingly to avoid pain or discomfort.

- Feel free to modify the exercise by performing it seated or lying down if standing is challenging for you.

Hip circles can be incorporated into your warm-up routine, as a break during prolonged sitting, or as part of a larger somatic exercise practice. They can help improve hip mobility, relieve stiffness, and promote a sense of ease and relaxation in the hips and pelvis. As always, if you have any specific concerns or underlying medical conditions, it's advisable to consult with a healthcare professional before starting any new exercise program.

Psoas Release

The psoas muscle is a deep hip flexor that connects the lower spine to the top of the thigh bone. It can become tight and tense due to prolonged sitting, stress, or physical activities. Releasing the psoas can help alleviate lower back pain, improve posture, and increase mobility in the hips and pelvis. Here's how to perform a Psoas Release:

- Lie down on your back on a comfortable surface, such as a yoga mat or carpet.

- Bend your knees and place your feet flat on the ground, hip-width apart.

- Take a few deep breaths to relax your body.

- Bring your attention to your right hip and imagine softening and releasing any tension in the area.

- Slowly bring your right knee towards your chest, hugging it gently.

- If comfortable, you can interlace your fingers and place them behind your right thigh to support the stretch.

- As you hold the stretch, continue to breathe deeply and relax.

- Stay in this position for about 1-2 minutes, allowing the psoas muscle to release.

- Repeat the same steps on the left side, bringing the left knee towards the chest.

- After completing both sides, you can extend your legs and rest for a few moments.

PELVIC CLOCK

The Pelvic Clock exercise is a somatic movement that helps improve awareness and mobility in the pelvis. It involves visualizing the pelvis as a clock face and moving it through various positions. Here's how to perform the Pelvic Clock exercise:

- Lie down on your back with your knees bent and feet flat on the ground, hip-width apart.

- Take a few deep breaths to relax your body and center your attention.

- Imagine that your pelvis is the center of a clock face.

- Start by tilting your pelvis forward, as if the clock hands are moving towards 12 o'clock.

- Return to the neutral position and then tilt your pelvis backward, as if the clock hands are moving towards 6 o'clock.

- Next, tilt your pelvis to the right side, as if the clock hands are moving towards 3 o'clock.

- Return to the neutral position and then tilt your pelvis to the left side, as if the clock hands are moving towards 9 o'clock.

- Continue to move your pelvis through these four positions, imagining a smooth, circular motion.

- As you perform the exercise, focus on the sensations in your pelvis and aim for smooth, controlled movements.

- Repeat the Pelvic Clock exercise for several rounds, allowing your pelvis to move freely and naturally.

Both the Psoas Release and Pelvic Clock exercises can be beneficial for promoting mobility, releasing tension, and improving awareness in the hips and pelvis. It's important to perform these exercises mindfully and listen to your body's feedback. If you have any specific concerns or underlying medical conditions, it's advisable to consult with a healthcare professional before starting any new exercise program.

Some additional information about the Psoas Release and Pelvic Clock exercises:

1. Psoas Release:

The psoas muscle is a deep hip flexor that runs from the lower spine through the pelvis and attaches to the top of the thigh bone. It plays a crucial role in stabilizing the spine, supporting posture, and facilitating movement in the hips and pelvis. When the psoas becomes tight or tense, it can lead to discomfort, lower back pain, and limited mobility.

The Psoas Release exercise aims to release tension and lengthen the psoas muscle. By gently bringing the knee towards the chest, you create a stretch in the psoas and allow it to relax. Holding the stretch for a few minutes provides an opportunity for the muscle to release and return to its optimal length.

It's important to approach the Psoas Release exercise with gentleness and mindfulness. Avoid any movements or positions that cause pain or discomfort. If you experience any discomfort during the exercise or have a history of hip or back injuries, it's advisable to consult with a healthcare professional before attempting the exercise.

Pelvic Clock

The Pelvic Clock exercise is a somatic movement that focuses on improving awareness and mobility in the pelvis. It allows you to explore the different movements and positions of the pelvis, helping to release tension, improve coordination, and enhance overall mobility.

The exercise involves visualizing the pelvis as a clock face. By tilting the pelvis forward, backward, and to the sides, you engage different muscles and encourage a full range of motion in the pelvis. The Pelvic Clock exercise can help improve pelvic stability, enhance core strength, and promote better alignment and posture.

It's important to perform the Pelvic Clock exercise with awareness and control. Focus on the quality of movement rather than the quantity. The exercise should be performed slowly and smoothly, allowing the pelvis to move through each position without any jerking or forcing. If you experience any discomfort or pain during the exercise, modify the range of motion or consult with a healthcare professional.

Both the Psoas Release and Pelvic Clock exercises can be incorporated into your regular movement routine or as part of a somatic practice. They are particularly beneficial for individuals who spend long hours sitting or have a sedentary lifestyle, as they help counteract the effects of prolonged sitting and promote healthy movement in the hips and pelvis.

It's worth noting that somatic exercises like these are most effective when practiced regularly over time. Consistency and mindful attention to your body's feedback are key to reaping the benefits of these exercises.

HIP OPENER

Hip openers are a category of exercises and stretches that target the muscles and joints in the hips, helping to increase flexibility, release tension, and improve overall mobility. Here are a few examples of hip-opening exercises:

1. Butterfly Stretch:

- Sit on the floor with your legs bent and the soles of your feet together, allowing your knees to fall out to the sides.

- Hold onto your ankles or feet with your hands.

- Keeping your spine straight, gently press your elbows against your inner thighs, encouraging a deeper stretch.

- Hold the stretch for 30 seconds to 1 minute while taking slow, deep breaths.

- To increase the intensity of the stretch, gently lean forward from your hips while maintaining a straight spine.

2. Pigeon Pose:

- Start in a high plank position, then slide your right knee forward towards your right hand, placing it on the ground behind your right wrist.

- Extend your left leg straight back behind you, keeping your hips squared to the front.

- Slowly lower your upper body down towards the ground, resting on your forearms or hands, while keeping your hips level.

- Hold the stretch for 30 seconds to 1 minute, then switch sides and repeat.

3. Lizard Lunge:

- Begin in a high plank position, then step your right foot forward and place it on the ground outside of your right hand.

- Lower your left knee to the ground and slide it back, so your left leg is extended behind you.

- Keep your hips squared to the front and sink your hips down towards the ground, feeling a stretch in your right hip flexor.

- You can stay on your hands or lower down onto your forearms for a deeper stretch.

- Hold the stretch for 30 seconds to 1 minute, then switch sides and repeat.

4. Standing Figure 4 Stretch:

- Stand with your feet hip-width apart.

- Lift your right foot off the ground and cross your right ankle over your left thigh, creating a figure 4 shape with your legs.

- Bend your left knee and lower your hips down into a squat position, keeping your chest lifted and your spine straight.

- You should feel a stretch in your right hip and glute area.

- Hold the stretch for 30 seconds to 1 minute, then switch sides and repeat.

It's important to approach hip-opening exercises with care and listen to your body. If you have any pre-existing hip injuries or conditions, it's advisable to consult with a healthcare professional before attempting these exercises. Start slowly, gradually increase the intensity, and always work within your comfortable range of motion. Remember to breathe deeply and relax into the stretches to maximize their benefits.

Chapter 6

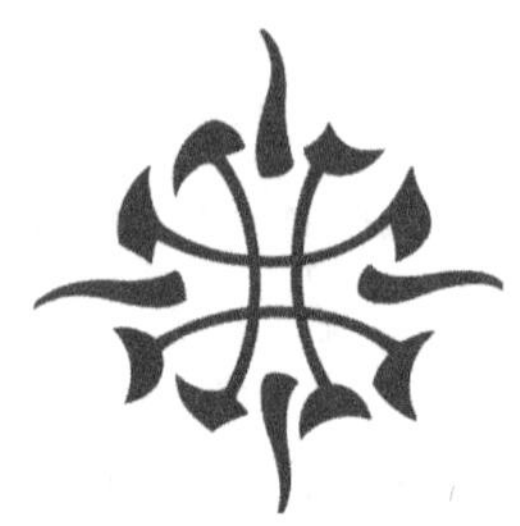

Somatic Exercises for the Legs and Feet

LEG SWINGS

Leg swings are a somatic exercise that targets the legs and feet, promoting mobility, flexibility, and improved circulation. They involve rhythmic swinging motions of the legs, which help to warm up the muscles, increase range of motion, and release tension. Here's how to perform leg swings:

1. Find a clear space where you have room to swing your legs without any obstructions.

2. Stand upright with your feet hip-width apart and engage your core muscles for stability.

3. Hold onto a wall, chair, or other support to maintain your balance if needed.

4. Begin with forward leg swings:

 - Shift your weight onto your right leg and allow your left leg to swing forward.

 - Swing your left leg as high as comfortable while keeping it straight or with a slight bend at the knee.

 - As your left leg swings forward, your right leg acts as a stabilizer.

 - Repeat the swinging motion for 10 to 15 swings on the left leg.

 - Switch to swinging your right leg forward and repeat the same number of swings.

5. After completing the forward leg swings, move on to lateral leg swings:

 - Stand perpendicular to a wall or support, with your left side facing the wall.

- Hold onto the wall or support with your left hand for balance.

- Swing your right leg out to the side, keeping it straight or with a slight bend at the knee.

- Swing your right leg across your body towards your left side, then swing it back out to the side.

- Repeat the swinging motion for 10 to 15 swings on the right leg.

- Turn to face the other direction and repeat the same number of swings on the left leg.

6. Finally, perform backward leg swings:

- Stand upright with your feet hip-width apart and your hands on your hips for support.

- Shift your weight onto your right leg and swing your left leg backward.

- Swing your left leg backward as high as comfortable while keeping it straight or with a slight bend at the knee.

- As your left leg swings backward, your right leg acts as a stabilizer.

- Repeat the swinging motion for 10 to 15 swings on the left leg.

- Switch to swinging your right leg backward and repeat the same number of swings.

7. Take a moment to stand still and notice any changes in your legs and feet. Pay attention to any sensations or areas of tension that may have been released.

8. Remember to perform the leg swings in a controlled manner, avoiding any jerking or forcing of the movements. Start with small swings and gradually increase the range of motion as your muscles warm up.

9. If you have any existing leg or foot injuries or conditions, it's advisable to consult with a healthcare professional before attempting leg swings or any other new exercise.

10. Leg swings can be incorporated into your warm-up routine before physical activity or used as a standalone exercise to improve leg and foot mobility. They can help increase blood flow, loosen up the muscles, and prepare your lower body for movement.

As with any exercise, listen to your body and modify the intensity or range of motion as needed. If you experience any pain or discomfort during leg swings, stop the exercise and consult a healthcare professional.

Somatic exercises focus on enhancing body awareness and promoting mindful movement. They can be beneficial for improving mobility, releasing tension, and increasing flexibility in the legs and feet. Here are a few additional somatic exercises for the lower body:

1. Calf Raises:

Calf raises target the calf muscles (gastrocnemius and soleus) and help strengthen the lower legs. Here's how to perform them:

- Stand with your feet hip-width apart, keeping your spine straight and shoulders relaxed.

- Slowly rise up onto the balls of your feet, lifting your heels as high as possible.

- Hold the raised position for a few seconds, then lower your heels back down to the ground.

- Repeat for 10 to 15 repetitions, gradually increasing the number as you become more comfortable.

2. Ankle Circles:

Ankle circles improve mobility and flexibility in the ankles and feet. Here's how to do them:

- Sit on a chair or the floor with your legs extended in front of you.

- Lift one foot off the ground and begin making circular motions with your ankle.

- Rotate your foot clockwise for several repetitions, then switch to counterclockwise rotations.

- Perform 10 to 15 circles in each direction, and then switch to the other foot.

3. Toe Spreading:

Toe spreading exercises help to strengthen the muscles in the feet and promote better foot alignment. Here's how to do them:

- Sit on a chair or the floor with your feet flat on the ground.

- Spread your toes apart as wide as possible, like you're trying to create space between them.

- Hold the spread for a few seconds, then relax your toes.

- Repeat for 10 to 15 repetitions, gradually increasing the duration and number of repetitions.

4. Standing Hamstring Stretch:

The standing hamstring stretch targets the hamstrings, which are the muscles at the back of the thighs. Here's how to perform it:

- Stand with your feet hip-width apart and take a step forward with your right foot.

- Keep your right leg straight and hinge forward at the hips, reaching towards your right toes.

- You should feel a stretch in the back of your right thigh.

- Hold the stretch for 20 to 30 seconds, then switch to the other leg.

Remember to approach these exercises with mindfulness and respect for your body's limitations. Start with gentle movements and gradually increase the intensity and range of motion as your body allows. If you have any pre-existing conditions or concerns, it's advisable to consult with a healthcare professional before attempting these exercises.

Incorporating somatic exercises for the legs and feet into your routine can help improve flexibility, reduce muscle tension, and enhance overall lower body function. They can be performed as standalone exercises or as part of a broader movement or stretching routine. Regular practice and consistency are key to experiencing the benefits of these exercises.

ANKLE ROLLS

Ankle rolls are a simple yet effective exercise for promoting ankle mobility and flexibility. They help to improve circulation, release tension, and enhance the range of motion in the ankles. Here's how to perform ankle rolls:

- Sit on a chair or the floor with your legs extended in front of you or stand with your feet hip-width apart.

- Lift one foot off the ground and rotate your ankle in a circular motion.

- Start by moving your ankle clockwise, making smooth and controlled circles with your foot. Perform 5 to 10 rotations in this direction.

- Then, switch to counterclockwise rotations, again performing 5 to 10 circles.

- Repeat the exercise with the other foot, making sure to perform an equal number of rotations in each direction.

Ankle rolls can be performed as a warm-up exercise before physical activity or as a standalone exercise to increase ankle mobility and relieve stiffness. It's important to perform the movements gently and avoid any force or discomfort. If you have any ankle injuries or conditions, it's advisable to consult with a healthcare professional before attempting ankle rolls.

CALF STRETCH

Calf stretches target the muscles in the back of the lower legs, primarily the gastrocnemius and soleus muscles. These stretches help to improve flexibility, reduce muscle tightness, and prevent calf-related issues such as cramps and strains. Here's a simple calf stretch:

- Stand facing a wall or use a sturdy object for support, such as a chair or railing.

- Take a step back with your right foot and keep your right leg straight.

- Bend your left knee and lean forward, placing your hands on the wall or support for balance.

- You should feel a stretch in your right calf muscle.

- Hold the stretch for 20 to 30 seconds, then switch sides and repeat the stretch with your left leg.

- For a deeper stretch, you can slightly adjust the position of your feet or take a bigger step back.

Calf stretches can be incorporated into your warm-up routine before exercise or as a part of your post-workout stretching. It's important to listen to your body and avoid bouncing or jerking movements during the stretch. If you have any calf injuries or conditions, it's advisable to consult with a healthcare professional before attempting calf stretches.

Remember to breathe deeply and relax into the stretches. Regular practice of ankle rolls and calf stretches can help improve ankle mobility, reduce muscle tightness, and contribute to overall lower leg health.

Some additional information on ankle rolls and calf stretches:

Ankle Rolls

Ankle rolls are a simple exercise that can be done to promote ankle mobility and flexibility. They involve rotating the ankle in a circular motion, which helps to increase joint range of motion and improve circulation in the area. Here are some key points to keep in mind when performing ankle rolls:

- You can perform ankle rolls while sitting on a chair or on the floor with your legs extended, or you can stand with your feet hip-width apart.

- Lift one foot off the ground and start by moving your ankle in a clockwise direction, making smooth and controlled circles with your foot.

- Gradually increase the size of the circles as you feel more comfortable, but be sure to maintain control throughout the movement.

- After completing several rotations in one direction, switch to counterclockwise rotations and perform an equal number of circles.

- Repeat the exercise with the other foot, ensuring that you perform an equal number of rotations in each direction.

Ankle rolls are a great exercise to incorporate into your daily routine, especially if you spend a lot of time on your feet or if you have limited ankle mobility. They can be done at any time of the day and can help relieve ankle stiffness and discomfort.

Calf Stretch

Calf stretches are beneficial for increasing flexibility in the calf muscles, which include the gastrocnemius and soleus muscles. These stretches can help alleviate tightness and reduce the risk of calf injuries. Here's how to perform a basic calf stretch:

- Stand facing a wall or use a sturdy object, such as a chair or railing, for support.

- Take a step back with your right foot, keeping your right leg straight.

- Bend your left knee and lean forward, placing your hands on the wall or support for balance.

- You should feel a stretch in your right calf muscle.

- Hold the stretch for 20 to 30 seconds, breathing deeply and allowing the muscle to relax.

- Repeat the stretch with your left leg, stepping back with your left foot and bending your right knee.

To deepen the stretch, you can make some adjustments:

- Move your back foot farther away from the wall or support.

- Keep your back heel on the ground and your toes pointed forward as you lean forward.

- You can also try performing the stretch with a slightly bent knee to target different areas of the calf muscles.

Calf stretches are particularly useful for individuals who engage in activities that put a lot of strain on the calves, such as running or jumping. They can be done as part of a warm-up routine before exercise or as a standalone stretch to relieve tightness after physical activity.

It's important to note that everyone's flexibility and range of motion may vary, so it's essential to listen to your body and avoid pushing yourself into any painful or uncomfortable positions. If you have any specific concerns or conditions related to your ankles or calves, it's best to consult with a healthcare professional or a qualified exercise specialist for personalized guidance.

Regular practice of ankle rolls and calf stretches can help improve ankle mobility, reduce muscle tightness, and contribute to overall lower leg health. Remember to start slowly and gradually increase the intensity or duration of the exercises over time.

TOE POINT AND FLEX

Toe point and flex exercises are simple movements that can help improve flexibility and strength in the muscles of the feet and toes. These exercises are commonly used in dance, gymnastics, and other activities that require precise footwork. Here's how to perform toe point and flex exercises:

1. Toe Point:

- Sit on a chair or the floor with your legs extended in front of you.

- Keep your back straight and shoulders relaxed.

- Start by pointing your toes away from your body, trying to create a straight line with your foot.

- Focus on pointing from the ankle joint and lengthening the toes.

- Hold the pointed position for a few seconds, feeling the stretch in the top of your foot.

- Release the point and relax your foot.

- Repeat the exercise for several repetitions, gradually increasing the duration of the pointed position.

Toe pointing helps to stretch the muscles on the top of the foot and promote ankle flexibility. It can also improve the aesthetic appearance of the foot when performing certain movements or poses.

2. Toe Flex:

- Sit on a chair or the floor with your legs extended in front of you.

- Keep your back straight and shoulders relaxed.

- Start by flexing your toes back toward your body, as if you're trying to touch your toes to your shins.

- Focus on engaging the muscles on the bottom of your foot and feeling the stretch in the back of your calf.

- Hold the flexed position for a few seconds, maintaining tension in the foot.

- Release the flex and relax your foot.

- Repeat the exercise for several repetitions, gradually increasing the duration of the flexed position.

Toe flexing helps to stretch the calf muscles and strengthen the muscles on the bottom of the foot. It can also improve foot stability and control during movements that require pushing off the toes.

Both toe point and flex exercises can be performed as standalone exercises or as part of a broader foot and ankle strengthening routine. They can be done at any time of the day and are particularly beneficial for individuals who spend a lot of time on their feet or engage in activities that require precise footwork.

As with any exercise, it's important to listen to your body and avoid any movements that cause pain or discomfort. If you have any pre-existing foot or ankle conditions, it's advisable to consult with a healthcare professional or a qualified exercise specialist for personalized guidance.

Regular practice of toe point and flex exercises can help improve foot flexibility, strength, and control. Start with gentle movements and gradually increase the intensity and duration over time.

Toe Point and Flex exercises are commonly used to improve foot and ankle mobility, strengthen the muscles of the feet, and enhance overall foot control and coordination. Here are some more details about these exercises:

Toe Point:

- Toe pointing involves extending the toes away from the body, creating a straight line with the foot. It primarily stretches the muscles on the top of the foot, such as the extensor hallucis longus and extensor digitorum longus.

- To perform a toe point, sit on a chair or the floor with your legs extended in front of you. Flex your ankles and then point your toes away from your body, lengthening the toes as much as possible.

- As you point your toes, try to maintain a straight line from the ankle to the tips of the toes. Hold the pointed position for a few seconds, feeling the stretch in the top of your foot.

- Repeat the exercise for several repetitions, gradually increasing the duration of the pointed position each time.

Toe Flex:

- Toe flexing involves pulling the toes back towards the body, as if trying to touch them to the shins. This primarily stretches the calf muscles (gastrocnemius and soleus) and strengthens the muscles on the bottom of the foot, such as the flexor hallucis longus and flexor digitorum longus.

- To perform a toe flex, sit on a chair or the floor with your legs extended in front of you. Point your toes away from your body, and then flex them back towards your shins, pulling the top of the foot towards you.

- Focus on engaging the muscles on the bottom of your foot and feeling the stretch in the back of your calf. Hold the flexed position for a few seconds.

- Repeat the exercise for several repetitions, gradually increasing the duration of the flexed position each time.

Toe point and flex exercises can be done as part of a warm-up routine before physical activity, as a standalone exercise to improve foot mobility and strength, or as a cool-down stretch after exercise. They are particularly beneficial for dancers, gymnasts, and athletes who rely on precise footwork and toe control.

It's important to perform these exercises with control and avoid any movements that cause pain or discomfort. If you have any foot or ankle injuries or conditions, it's advisable to consult with a healthcare professional or a qualified exercise specialist for personalized guidance.

Incorporating regular toe point and flex exercises into your routine can help improve foot flexibility, strengthen foot muscles, and enhance overall foot and ankle function. Gradually increase the intensity and duration of these exercises over time, and remember to listen to your body's feedback during the movements.

Chapter 7

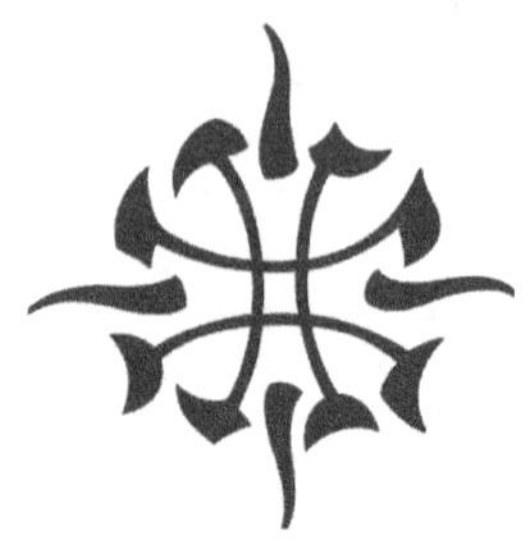

Somatic Exercises for Relaxation and Stress Relief

BREATHING EXERCISES

Somatic exercises can be great for relaxation and stress relief, and breathing exercises are particularly effective for calming the mind and body. Here are some breathing exercises you can try:

1. Deep Belly Breathing:

- Find a comfortable seated position or lie down on your back.

- Place one hand on your chest and the other on your abdomen.

- Take a slow, deep breath in through your nose, allowing your abdomen to rise as you fill your lungs with air.

- Exhale slowly through your mouth, feeling your abdomen gently fall as you release the breath.

- Continue deep belly breathing for several minutes, focusing on the sensation of your breath entering and leaving your body.

Deep belly breathing, also known as diaphragmatic breathing, helps activate the body's relaxation response and can promote a sense of calmness and relaxation.

2. 4-7-8 Breathing:

- Find a comfortable seated position.

- Close your eyes and take a few deep breaths to relax.

- Inhale quietly through your nose to a mental count of four.

- Hold your breath for a count of seven.

- Exhale slowly through your mouth to a count of eight.

- Repeat this cycle three more times, for a total of four breaths.

The 4-7-8 breathing technique is a simple and effective method for calming the nervous system and inducing a state of relaxation.

3. Box Breathing:

- Sit comfortably and take a few deep breaths to relax.

- Inhale slowly through your nose to a count of four, feeling your abdomen rise.

- Hold your breath for a count of four.

- Exhale slowly through your nose or mouth to a count of four.

- Hold your breath for a count of four before starting the next breath.

- Repeat this cycle for several minutes, focusing on the equal duration of each phase of the breath.

Box breathing is a technique commonly used in mindfulness and meditation practices to promote relaxation, reduce anxiety, and enhance mental clarity.

These breathing exercises can be done anytime, anywhere, and can be particularly helpful during moments of stress or when you need to relax and unwind. Regular practice of these exercises can improve your ability to manage stress and promote a sense of calmness in your daily life.

Remember to breathe deeply, with slow and controlled breaths, and allow your body to relax with each exhalation. Feel free to adjust the duration of each phase of the breath to suit your comfort level.

In addition to breathing exercises, other somatic exercises for relaxation and stress relief include progressive muscle relaxation, body scans, and gentle stretching. It's important to find what works best for you and incorporate these practices into your routine as needed.

Please note that while these exercises can be beneficial for relaxation and stress relief, they are not a substitute for professional help or treatment for stress-related disorders. If you are experiencing chronic or severe stress, it's important to seek guidance from a healthcare professional or a qualified mental health practitioner.

PROGRESSIVE MUSCLE RELAXATION

Progressive Muscle Relaxation (PMR) is a technique that involves systematically tensing and releasing different muscle groups in the body to promote relaxation. Here's how you can practice PMR:

- Find a quiet and comfortable space where you can relax without distractions.

- Start by taking a few deep breaths to center yourself and bring your attention to the present moment.

- Begin with a specific muscle group, such as your hands or feet. Tense the muscles in that area for about 5-10 seconds, while maintaining deep breathing.

- After the tensing phase, release the tension completely and allow the muscles to relax for 15-20 seconds.

- Move on to the next muscle group, working your way through the body. You can progress from your feet to your legs, hips, abdomen, chest, arms, neck, and finally to your face and scalp.

- As you tense and release each muscle group, pay attention to the sensations of tension and relaxation. Focus on the contrast between the two states.

- Continue the process until you have gone through all major muscle groups or until you feel a deep sense of relaxation.

Progressive Muscle Relaxation helps to reduce muscle tension, release physical stress, and promote overall relaxation. It can be particularly beneficial for individuals who hold tension in specific areas of their body due to stress or anxiety.

Body Scan Meditation

Body scan meditation is a mindfulness practice that involves bringing focused attention to each part of the body, systematically scanning from head to toe. Here's how you can practice body scan meditation:

- Find a comfortable position, either sitting or lying down, with your eyes closed.

- Begin by bringing your attention to your breath, taking a few deep breaths to relax.

- Slowly direct your attention to the sensations in your body, starting with the top of your head.

- Gradually move your attention down through each part of your body, paying attention to any sensations, tension, or areas of discomfort.

- As you scan each body part, try to soften and relax any areas of tension or tightness that you become aware of.

- Stay present with each part of your body, observing the sensations without judgment or the need to change anything.

- Continue scanning down to your toes, bringing awareness to your entire body.

- If your mind wanders, gently guide your attention back to the body part you were focusing on.

- Take a few moments to feel the overall sense of relaxation and calmness in your body.

Body scan meditation helps to cultivate a sense of mindfulness and body awareness, allowing you to connect with the present moment and release tension held in the body. It can contribute to a greater sense of relaxation and well-being.

Both progressive muscle relaxation and body scan meditation can be practiced regularly to promote relaxation, reduce stress, and increase overall body awareness. They can be done independently or as part of a larger relaxation or mindfulness routine.

Remember that these exercises are not intended to replace professional treatment for stress-related conditions. If you are experiencing chronic or severe stress, it's important to seek guidance from a healthcare professional or a qualified mental health practitioner.

Here is some additional information on progressive muscle relaxation and body scan motivation:

Progressive Muscle Relaxation

Progressive Muscle Relaxation (PMR) was developed by American physician Edmund Jacobson in the early 20th century. It is based on the principle that tensing and then releasing specific muscle groups can promote deep relaxation and reduce muscle tension.

The technique is effective because it helps individuals become more aware of the physical sensations of tension and relaxation in their bodies. By deliberately tensing and then releasing the muscles, you can learn to differentiate between the two states and develop a greater sense of control over your muscle tension.

Progressive Muscle Relaxation has been widely used to manage stress, anxiety, and insomnia. It can also be helpful for individuals experiencing chronic pain, headaches, or muscle-related tension disorders.

In addition to promoting relaxation, PMR has been found to have other benefits, including:

- **Improved sleep quality:** Practicing PMR before bedtime can help calm the mind and body, making it easier to fall asleep and experience more restful sleep.

- **Stress reduction:** By consciously releasing muscle tension, PMR can lower overall stress levels and promote a sense of calmness.

- **Enhanced body awareness:** PMR helps cultivate a greater awareness of the body, enabling individuals to recognize and address areas of muscle tension or discomfort.

Progressive Muscle Relaxation is a skill that can be learned and practiced independently or guided by a trained professional. Guided audio recordings or apps can provide step-by-step instructions to assist with the practice.

Body Scan Meditation

Body scan meditation is a mindfulness practice that involves systematically directing attention to different parts of the body, from head to toe or vice versa. The purpose is to cultivate a non-judgmental awareness of bodily sensations, thoughts, and emotions that arise in each moment.

The practice of body scan meditation can vary, but here's a general outline:

- Find a quiet and comfortable place to sit or lie down, where you won't be disturbed.

- Close your eyes and take a few deep breaths to center yourself.

- Begin by bringing your attention to the top of your head and gradually move downward, observing sensations in each body part as you go along.

- Notice any physical sensations, such as warmth, coolness, tingling, or tension. Also, be aware of any thoughts or emotions that arise.

- If you come across areas of tension or discomfort, you can bring a sense of softness and relaxation to those areas by directing your breath and attention there.

- Practice non-judgmental observation, simply noticing the sensations without trying to change them or attaching any labels.

- Continue the scan until you reach the tips of your toes or complete the cycle from head to toe.

Body scan meditation helps develop a deep connection between the mind and body and cultivates a sense of present-moment awareness. It allows individuals to observe physical sensations and mental states with curiosity and acceptance.

Research has shown that regular practice of body scan meditation can have several benefits, including:

- Stress reduction: Body scan meditation helps to activate the relaxation response, promoting a sense of calm and reducing stress levels.

- Increased body awareness: By paying attention to the body, individuals can develop a greater awareness of their physical sensations and gain insights into their overall well-being.

- Mind-body integration: The practice helps bridge the gap between the mind and body, fostering a greater sense of wholeness and unity.

Body scan meditation can be practiced independently or guided by a meditation app, audio recording, or a meditation teacher. It is often included as a component of mindfulness-based stress reduction (MBSR) programs.

Remember that both progressive muscle relaxation and body scan meditation are practices that require regularity and patience. With consistent practice, they can become valuable tools for relaxation, stress management, and overall well-being.

GUIDED IMAGERY

Guided imagery is another somatic exercise that can be used for relaxation and stress relief. It involves using the power of imagination and visualization to create a mental experience that promotes relaxation and well-being. Here's an overview of guided imagery:

Guided imagery is a practice that involves using your imagination to create vivid mental images and scenarios that evoke a sense of calmness, relaxation, and well-being. It can be done with the help of a guided meditation recording, an instructor, or by following a script.

Here's how you can practice guided imagery:

- Find a quiet and comfortable space where you can relax without interruptions.

- Close your eyes and take a few deep breaths to settle your mind and body.

- Choose a specific theme or scenario for your guided imagery practice. It can be a peaceful nature scene, a favorite place from your past, or any soothing scenario that resonates with you.

- Begin to vividly imagine the details of the scene using all your senses. Visualize the colors, shapes, and textures. Imagine any sounds, smells, or tastes associated with the scene.

- As you immerse yourself in the imagery, allow yourself to experience a sense of relaxation and well-being. Focus on the positive emotions and sensations that arise.

- If distracting thoughts arise, gently bring your attention back to the imagery and the feelings it evokes.

- You can continue to explore the scene and deepen your experience for as long as you wish.

- When you're ready to end the practice, gradually bring your awareness back to the present moment. Take a few deep breaths and slowly open your eyes.

Guided imagery can be a powerful tool for relaxation and stress relief. It taps into the mind's ability to create a mental experience that can positively influence the body's physiological response, promoting a state of calmness and relaxation.

Research has shown that guided imagery can have various benefits, including:

- Stress reduction: Imagining peaceful and calming scenes can help reduce stress levels and activate the relaxation response in the body.

- Anxiety management: Guided imagery can be effective in reducing anxiety symptoms and promoting a greater sense of calm and control.

- Pain management: Imagery techniques have been used to alleviate pain and improve overall well-being in individuals with chronic pain conditions.

- Enhancing performance: Guided imagery has been used by athletes, musicians, and performers to enhance focus, confidence, and performance.

Guided imagery can be practiced independently using pre-recorded audio tracks, apps, or guided meditation scripts. You can also seek the guidance of a trained instructor or therapist who specializes in imagery techniques.

It's important to note that guided imagery is a complementary practice and should not replace professional medical or mental health care. If you have specific concerns or conditions, it's advisable to consult with a healthcare professional who can guide you in the appropriate use of guided imagery for your specific needs.

Chapter 8

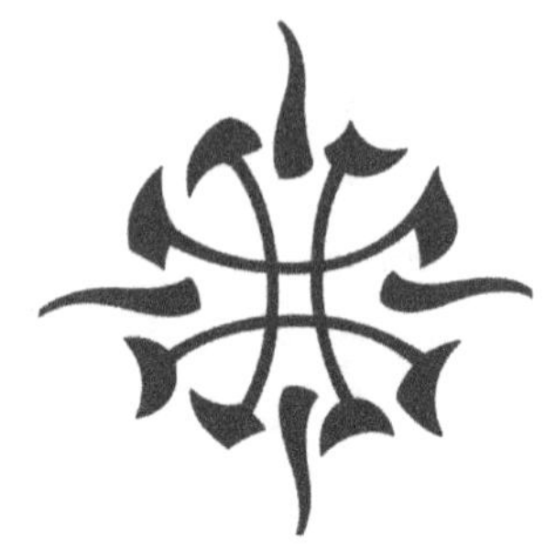

Building a Somatic Exercise Routine

Creating a Personal Practice Plan

Building a somatic exercise routine can be a valuable way to incorporate relaxation, stress relief, and overall well-being into your daily life. Here are some steps to help you create a personal practice plan:

1. Set your goals: Start by clarifying what you hope to achieve through your somatic exercise routine. It could be stress reduction, relaxation, increased body awareness, improved sleep, or any other specific outcome. Having clear goals will help you design a practice that aligns with your intentions.

2. Choose somatic exercises: Consider the somatic exercises that resonate with you and align with your goals. You can include a combination of progressive muscle relaxation, body scan meditation, guided imagery, and other techniques that you find beneficial. Select exercises that you enjoy and that suit your preferences and needs.

3. Determine frequency and duration: Decide how often you would like to practice your somatic exercises. It can be daily, a few times a week, or as per your schedule and availability. Also, consider the duration of each practice session. Start with a realistic timeframe, such as 10-15 minutes, and adjust it based on your comfort and time constraints.

4. Create a schedule: Establish a regular schedule for your somatic exercise routine. Choose a time of day when you can dedicate uninterrupted time for your practice. Consistency is key, so try to stick to your schedule as much as possible. You can also set reminders or incorporate your routine into your existing daily rituals.

5. Find a quiet and comfortable space: Identify a quiet and comfortable space where you can practice your somatic exercises without distractions. It could be a designated room, a corner of your home, or any place where you can relax and focus without interruptions.

6. Start with a warm-up: Consider incorporating a brief warm-up at the beginning of your routine. This can include gentle stretching, deep breathing, or any other activity that helps you transition into a relaxed state and prepares your body and mind for the somatic exercises.

7. Mix and match: Keep your routine varied and engaging by incorporating different somatic exercises. You can alternate between progressive muscle relaxation, body scan meditation, guided imagery, and even explore other mindfulness practices such as deep breathing exercises or gentle yoga poses. This variety can help prevent boredom and maintain your interest.

8. Seek guidance if needed: If you're new to somatic exercises or want to deepen your practice, consider seeking guidance from a trained instructor or using guided audio recordings or apps. They can provide structure, guidance, and support as you develop your routine.

9. Listen to your body: Pay attention to your body's signals and adjust your practice accordingly. If a particular exercise feels uncomfortable or causes pain, modify it or seek guidance from a professional. Your somatic exercise routine should be gentle, enjoyable, and supportive of your overall well-being.

10. Track your progress: Keep a journal or record of your somatic exercise practice. Note any changes or benefits you experience over time. This can help you stay motivated, track your progress, and reflect on the positive impact of your routine.

Remember that consistency and patience are important when developing a somatic exercise routine. It may take time to fully experience the benefits, so be gentle with yourself and trust the process.

Additionally, it's worth mentioning that somatic exercises can be a valuable complement to other self-care practices, such as maintaining a healthy lifestyle, getting sufficient sleep, and seeking support from professionals when needed.

Feel free to adapt and modify your routine as you go along to suit your evolving needs and preferences. Enjoy the journey of exploring somatic exercises and discovering the positive impact they can have on your well-being.

Combining Exercises and Sequencing

Combining different somatic exercises and sequencing them in a thoughtful manner can enhance the effectiveness and variety of your practice. Here are some considerations for combining exercises and creating a sequence:

1. Start with a centering practice: Begin your sequence with a centering exercise, such as deep breathing or a brief mindfulness meditation. This helps you transition from your daily activities into a focused and present state of mind.

2. Choose complementary exercises: Select exercises that complement each other and align with your goals. For example, you can combine progressive muscle relaxation with body scan meditation to promote both relaxation and body awareness. Consider how each exercise can build upon or enhance the benefits of the previous one.

3. Gradual progression: Structure your sequence in a way that allows for a gradual progression. Start with exercises that are more accessible and easier to practice, and then gradually move on to more challenging ones. This helps you build skills, deepen your practice, and avoid overwhelming yourself.

4. Balance relaxation and activation: Include a balance of relaxation-focused exercises and those that promote activation and energization. This can help you achieve a well-rounded practice that addresses both physical tension and mental alertness.

5. Mind-body integration: Integrate exercises that focus on both the mind and body. For example, you can combine guided imagery with progressive muscle relaxation to engage both your imagination and physical sensations. This fosters a deeper mind-body connection and enhances the overall experience.

6. Consider time constraints: Be mindful of the time available for your practice and create a sequence that fits within that timeframe. If you have limited time, prioritize the exercises that are most beneficial for you and adjust the duration accordingly.

7. Personal preferences: Take into account your personal preferences and what resonates with you. If you find a particular exercise more enjoyable or effective, give it more emphasis in your sequence. Tailor the sequence to suit your individual needs and preferences.

8. Smooth transitions: Ensure that the transitions between exercises are smooth and seamless. Take a moment of pause or deep breaths between exercises to allow yourself to fully transition and integrate the benefits of each exercise.

PROGRESSION AND CHALLENGE

As you become more comfortable with your somatic exercise routine, you may want to introduce progression and challenge to further deepen your practice. Here are some ways to progress and challenge yourself:

1. Longer practice sessions: Gradually increase the duration of your practice sessions to allow for more exploration and immersion in the exercises. This can help you develop a greater capacity for relaxation and focus.

2. Intensify muscle tension and release: When practicing progressive muscle relaxation, experiment with gradually increasing the level of muscle tension during the "tensing" phase and then fully releasing the tension during the "relaxation" phase. This can help you develop greater awareness of muscle tension and relaxation.

3. Explore different body scan variations: Expand your body scan meditation practice by exploring different variations. You can try focusing on specific areas of the body that require attention or incorporating mindfulness of breath alongside the body scan. This deepens your ability to observe and explore bodily sensations.

4. Experiment with advanced guided imagery: If you're comfortable with guided imagery, explore more advanced scenarios or themes that challenge your imagination and visualization skills. This can include more complex landscapes, journeys, or narratives that require deeper engagement.

5. Incorporate movement: Consider integrating gentle movement or mindful yoga poses into your somatic exercise routine. This adds a dynamic element to your practice and promotes a greater sense of embodiment.

6. Seek professional guidance: If you feel ready for a deeper challenge or want to refine your practice, consider seeking guidance from a somatic practitioner, meditation teacher, or therapist. They can provide personalized guidance, introduce advanced techniques, and support your progress.

Remember to listen to your body and adjust the level of challenge based on your comfort and abilities. It's important to maintain a balance between gentle progression and avoiding pushing yourself beyond your limits.

By combining exercises thoughtfully and gradually introducing challenges, you can continually deepen your somatic exercise practice and experience the benefits on a deeper level.

Feel free to adapt and modify your sequence and level of challenge based on your own preferences and progress. It's your personal practice, and you have the flexibility to customize it to suit your needs and growth.

Chapter 9

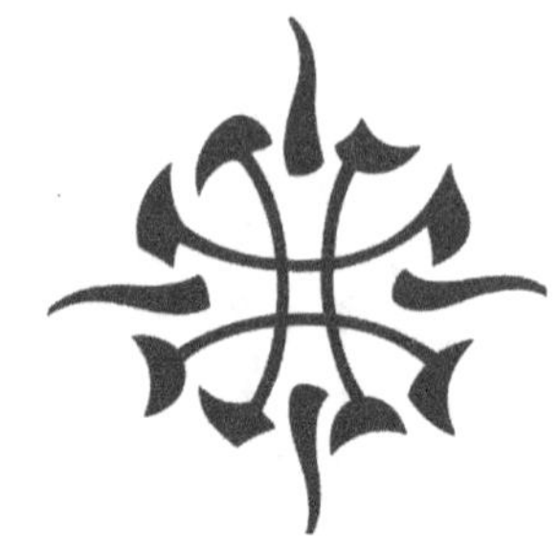

Frequently Asked Questions (FAQs)

COMMON CONCERNS AND MISCONCEPTIONS

Somatic exercises and practices can sometimes raise questions or create misconceptions. Here are some common concerns and misconceptions addressed:

Q1: Are somatic exercises only for people with physical ailments or injuries?

A1: No, somatic exercises can benefit anyone, regardless of their physical condition. While they can be helpful for managing pain or recovering from injuries, somatic practices are also valuable for stress reduction, relaxation, body awareness, and overall well-being.

Q2: Can somatic exercises replace medical or mental health treatments?

A2: Somatic exercises can be a valuable complement to medical or mental health treatments, but they should not replace professional care. If you have specific medical or mental health concerns, it's important to consult with appropriate healthcare professionals for diagnosis and treatment.

Q3: Do I need prior experience or special skills to practice somatic exercises?

A3: No, prior experience or special skills are not necessary. Somatic exercises are accessible to everyone, regardless of their background. They are designed to be gentle, simple, and suitable for beginners. With regular practice and patience, you can develop and deepen your skills over time.

Q4: Can somatic exercises be practiced by older adults or individuals with limited mobility?

A4: Yes, somatic exercises can be adapted for individuals of all ages and abilities. They can be modified to accommodate physical limitations or mobility challenges. It's important to work within your comfort level and consult with a healthcare professional or somatic practitioner if needed.

Q5: How long does it take to experience the benefits of somatic exercises?

A5: The benefits of somatic exercises can vary from person to person. Some individuals may experience immediate relaxation and stress relief after a single session, while others may require consistent practice over a period of time to notice significant changes. Regular practice and patience are key to experiencing the long-term benefits.

Q6: Can somatic exercises be practiced during pregnancy?

A6: Somatic exercises can be beneficial during pregnancy, but it's important to consult with a healthcare provider before starting or modifying any exercise routine. Certain exercises may need to be adapted or avoided based on individual circumstances or trimesters.

Q7: Can somatic exercises be practiced with children?

A7: Yes, somatic exercises can be adapted for children. However, it's important to consider age-appropriate exercises and engage children in a way that is enjoyable and suitable for their developmental stage. It can be helpful to seek guidance from professionals who specialize in somatic practices for children.

Q8: Are somatic exercises religious or spiritual in nature?

A8: Somatic exercises are not inherently religious or spiritual. While mindfulness or meditation practices may have roots in certain spiritual traditions, somatic exercises themselves can be secular and focused on promoting relaxation, body awareness, and well-being. They can be practiced in a way that aligns with your personal beliefs and values.

Remember that these answers provide general information, and individual experiences may vary. It's always recommended to consult with healthcare professionals or somatic practitioners for personalized guidance and support.

TROUBLESHOOTING TIPS

Sometimes, you may encounter challenges or difficulties when practicing somatic exercises. Here are some troubleshooting tips to help you navigate common issues:

1. Lack of focus or distractions: If you find it challenging to stay focused during your somatic exercise practice, try practicing in a quiet and dedicated space, free from distractions. Consider using headphones to listen to guided audio recordings that can help keep your attention engaged.

2. Physical discomfort or pain: Somatic exercises should be gentle and comfortable. If you experience physical discomfort or pain during an exercise, modify it to suit your needs or seek guidance from a somatic practitioner or healthcare professional. It's important to listen to your body and avoid pushing beyond your limits.

3. Difficulty relaxing or letting go of tension: Relaxation can take time, especially if you're dealing with chronic stress or tension. Practice patience and persistence. Experiment with different relaxation techniques, such as deep breathing or progressive muscle relaxation, to find what works best for you. Regular practice can help train your body and mind to relax more easily.

4. Feeling overwhelmed or anxious: If you feel overwhelmed or anxious during your somatic exercise practice, take a moment to pause, breathe, and ground yourself. Start with shorter practice sessions and gradually increase the duration as you become more comfortable. If needed, seek support from a mental health professional who can provide guidance and help you manage anxiety or other emotional challenges.

5. Lack of motivation or consistency: If you're struggling to maintain motivation or consistency, remind yourself of the benefits you've experienced or the goals you've set. Consider finding an accountability partner or joining a somatic exercise class or group to stay motivated. Breaking your routine into smaller, manageable chunks can also help maintain consistency.